Table Of Contents

Chapter 1: Understanding Osteoporosis

What is Osteoporosis?

Osteoporosis is a progressive bone disease characterized by decreased bone density and strength, which increases the risk of fractures. It often develops silently over many years, making it difficult for individuals to recognize its presence until a fracture occurs. The condition is particularly prevalent among postmenopausal women due to the significant drop in estrogen levels, which plays a crucial role in maintaining bone density. However, osteoporosis can also affect men and children, highlighting the importance of awareness and education across all demographics.

The underlying cause of osteoporosis is an imbalance between bone resorption and bone formation. In healthy individuals, these processes are finely tuned, ensuring that bone density remains stable. However, various factors, including aging, hormonal changes, nutritional deficiencies, and certain chronic diseases, can disrupt this balance. Particularly in postmenopausal women, the decline in estrogen leads to increased bone resorption, resulting in a net loss of bone mass. In children, conditions such as juvenile idiopathic arthritis or prolonged corticosteroid use can lead to pediatric osteoporosis, emphasizing that this condition is not limited to older adults.

Nutrition plays a critical role in bone health, as adequate intake of calcium, vitamin D, and other nutrients is essential for maintaining bone density. Calcium is vital for bone formation, while vitamin D facilitates calcium absorption in the gut. Deficiencies in these nutrients can significantly contribute to the development of osteoporosis. Moreover, certain lifestyle choices, such as excessive alcohol consumption and smoking, can further weaken bones. Therefore, a well-balanced diet combined with healthy lifestyle choices is crucial for both prevention and management of osteoporosis.

Screening and diagnosis of osteoporosis typically involve bone density tests, such as dual-energy X-ray absorptiometry (DEXA), which measure bone mineral density (BMD). These assessments help identify individuals at risk of fractures, allowing for early intervention. Understanding personal risk factors, including family history, age, gender, and lifestyle habits, is essential for effective screening. Regular check-ups and discussions with healthcare providers can facilitate timely diagnosis and management, thereby reducing the likelihood of osteoporotic fractures.

Osteoporotic fractures, particularly in the hip, spine, and wrist, can lead to significant morbidity and reduced quality of life. Rehabilitation following such fractures often involves a multidisciplinary approach, including physical therapy and exercise programs designed to strengthen muscles and improve balance. Furthermore, medications such as bisphosphonates or hormone replacement therapy may be prescribed to help manage the condition. Emphasizing prevention strategies, such as regular weight-bearing exercise and ensuring adequate nutrition, can empower patients to take an active role in managing their bone health and reducing the risk of fractures.

Risk Factors for Osteoporosis

Risk factors for osteoporosis can be broadly categorized into non-modifiable and modifiable factors. Non-modifiable factors include age, gender, and family history. As individuals age, bone density naturally decreases, making older adults particularly susceptible to osteoporosis. Women are at a higher risk, especially postmenopausal women, due to the significant drop in estrogen levels that occurs during menopause. This hormonal change accelerates bone loss, increasing the likelihood of developing osteoporosis. A family history of osteoporosis can also elevate an individual's risk, suggesting a genetic predisposition that may affect bone health.

Modifiable risk factors encompass lifestyle choices and health conditions that can be altered to improve bone health. Nutrition plays a crucial role; inadequate intake of calcium and vitamin D can lead to decreased bone density. Calcium is essential for bone formation, while vitamin D helps the body absorb calcium effectively. Furthermore, excessive alcohol consumption and smoking are detrimental to bone health. Alcohol can interfere with the body's ability to absorb nutrients necessary for bone maintenance, while smoking has been linked to reduced bone density and increased fracture risk.

Certain medical conditions can also contribute to the development of osteoporosis. Chronic diseases such as rheumatoid arthritis, gastrointestinal diseases, and hyperthyroidism can impact bone health. Medications used to treat these conditions, particularly corticosteroids, can also lead to bone density loss over time. It is important for patients to discuss their medical history and any medications they are taking with their healthcare provider to assess their individual risk for osteoporosis and explore potential alternatives or protective measures.

Physical inactivity is another modifiable risk factor affecting bone health. Weight-bearing and resistance exercises are essential for maintaining bone density and promoting overall musculoskeletal strength. A sedentary lifestyle can lead to a decrease in bone strength, making individuals more prone to fractures. Incorporating regular physical activity into daily routines is vital for osteoporosis prevention and management, especially for those identified as at risk.

Lastly, understanding the interplay between osteoporosis and other chronic diseases is essential for effective management. Conditions such as diabetes, chronic obstructive pulmonary disease (COPD), and kidney disease can exacerbate bone loss and increase fracture risk. It is crucial for patients with these conditions to work closely with their healthcare providers to monitor bone health and implement strategies that address both their chronic conditions and their osteoporosis risk factors. By recognizing and managing these risk factors, patients can take proactive steps toward maintaining strong bones and reducing their likelihood of osteoporotic fractures.

Symptoms and Complications

Osteoporosis is often referred to as a silent disease because it can progress without noticeable symptoms until a fracture occurs. Many individuals with osteoporosis may not realize they have weakened bones until they experience a significant injury. Common signs may include a sudden onset of back pain, which can indicate a spinal fracture, or a noticeable decrease in height over time due to vertebral compression. These symptoms highlight the importance of proactive screening and diagnosis, particularly in high-risk populations such as postmenopausal women and older adults.

In addition to fractures, osteoporosis can lead to a range of complications that significantly impact quality of life. Osteoporotic fractures, particularly in the hip, wrist, and spine, can result in severe pain, reduced mobility, and even loss of independence. Hip fractures are particularly concerning, as they often require surgical intervention and can lead to prolonged rehabilitation or complications such as deep vein thrombosis and pulmonary embolism. Understanding these risks is crucial for patients to take preventive measures and seek timely medical advice.

Pediatric osteoporosis, though less common, can also present unique symptoms and complications. Children with this condition may experience fractures from relatively minor falls or injuries, which can lead to ongoing pain and limitations in physical activity. The psychological impact of living with osteoporosis at a young age can also be significant, potentially affecting self-esteem and social interactions. It is vital for caregivers and healthcare providers to recognize these symptoms early to implement effective management strategies.

Nutrition plays a crucial role in bone health, and deficiencies in key nutrients can exacerbate osteoporosis symptoms. For instance, insufficient calcium and vitamin D intake can lead to further deterioration of bone density. Patients should be aware of the signs of nutritional deficiencies, such as fatigue, muscle weakness, and bone pain. Incorporating a balanced diet rich in these nutrients, alongside appropriate supplementation, can help mitigate symptoms and support overall bone health.

Complications from osteoporosis extend beyond physical limitations. The psychological effects of living with a chronic condition can lead to anxiety and depression, particularly following a fracture. Patients may fear future injuries, leading to decreased physical activity and social withdrawal. Addressing these emotional aspects is essential for comprehensive management. Seeking support from healthcare professionals, engaging in community resources, and participating in exercise programs tailored for osteoporosis can improve both physical and mental well-being, ultimately enhancing the quality of life for those affected.

Chapter 2: Osteoporosis in Postmenopausal Women

Hormonal Changes and Bone Health

Hormonal changes have a profound impact on bone health, particularly during critical life stages such as puberty, pregnancy, and menopause. Estrogen and testosterone, key hormones in the body, play significant roles in maintaining bone density. In women, the decline in estrogen levels during menopause leads to an increase in bone resorption, which can result in a rapid loss of bone mass.

This loss can significantly heighten the risk of developing osteoporosis, making it essential for postmenopausal women to understand the relationship between hormones and bone health.

In pediatric populations, hormonal changes occur during puberty, leading to rapid bone growth and increased bone density. The surge in growth hormones, along with sex hormones, contributes to the development of strong bones during this critical period. However, any disruption in hormone levels, whether due to health conditions or nutritional deficiencies, can adversely affect bone development and may predispose children to osteoporosis later in life. Ensuring adequate nutrition and physical activity during these formative years is crucial in fostering optimal bone health.

Men also experience hormonal changes that can impact bone density. Testosterone plays a vital role in maintaining bone strength in men. As men age, testosterone levels gradually decline, which can contribute to a decrease in bone density and an increased risk of osteoporosis. Understanding the signs of low testosterone and seeking appropriate medical evaluation can help men take proactive steps in managing their bone health and mitigating the risk of fractures associated with osteoporosis.

Nutrition is an essential element in the context of hormonal changes and bone health. Key nutrients such as calcium and vitamin D are crucial for bone formation and maintenance, particularly during periods of hormonal fluctuation. Postmenopausal women, for instance, may benefit from increased calcium intake to counteract the effects of declining estrogen levels. Additionally, incorporating foods rich in these nutrients, along with regular exercise, can enhance bone density and overall health. For pediatric patients, a diet that supports healthy hormonal development is equally important to ensure that bones reach their full potential in strength and density.

Lastly, the management of osteoporosis often involves hormone-related therapies, such as estrogen replacement therapy for postmenopausal women. These treatments can help mitigate bone loss and reduce the risk of fractures. However, it is essential for patients to discuss the potential benefits and risks associated with these therapies with their healthcare providers. Understanding how hormonal changes affect bone health empowers patients to make informed decisions about their osteoporosis management strategies, ensuring a proactive approach to maintaining strong bones throughout their lives.

Impact of Menopause on Bone Density

Menopause marks a significant transition in a woman's life, characterized by the end of menstrual cycles and a decline in reproductive hormones, particularly estrogen. This hormonal shift has profound implications for various bodily systems, including bone health. Estrogen plays a crucial role in maintaining bone density by inhibiting bone resorption, the process by which osteoclasts break down bone tissue. As estrogen levels decrease during and after menopause, women experience an accelerated rate of bone loss, which can lead to increased susceptibility to osteoporosis.

Research indicates that women can lose up to 20% of their bone density in the first five to seven years following menopause. This rapid decline is primarily due to the imbalance between bone resorption and bone formation. While the body continues to produce new bone tissue, the loss of estrogen means that this new bone is not being formed at a sufficient rate to counteract the increased resorption. Consequently, many women find themselves at a higher risk for osteoporotic fractures, particularly in the hip, spine, and wrist.

The impact of menopause on bone density is not uniform across all women; several factors can influence the extent of bone loss. Genetics, lifestyle choices, and overall health can all play a role in determining how significantly a woman may be affected. For instance, women with a family history of osteoporosis or those who are underweight may face higher risks. Additionally, lifestyle factors such as smoking, excessive alcohol consumption, and a sedentary lifestyle can exacerbate bone density loss during this critical period.

Preventive measures and interventions can help mitigate the risk of osteoporosis in postmenopausal women. Nutritional strategies, such as increasing calcium and vitamin D intake, are essential in supporting bone health. Weight-bearing exercises can also strengthen bones and improve balance, reducing the likelihood of falls and fractures. Furthermore, regular screenings for bone density can help identify women at risk, allowing for timely intervention through medications that may slow bone loss and promote bone formation.

In conclusion, understanding the impact of menopause on bone density is vital for women as they navigate this natural life stage. By recognizing the risks associated with declining estrogen levels and adopting proactive lifestyle changes, women can take significant steps toward preserving their bone health. Engaging with healthcare providers to discuss personalized strategies for prevention, treatment, and monitoring is essential in managing osteoporosis and fostering long-term well-being.

Strategies for Managing Osteoporosis in Postmenopausal Women

Managing osteoporosis in postmenopausal women requires a multifaceted approach that includes lifestyle modifications, nutritional strategies, medication adherence, and regular monitoring. Each of these components plays a vital role in maintaining bone health and preventing fractures. Understanding the significance of these strategies can empower patients to take control of their health, improve their quality of life, and minimize the risks associated with osteoporosis.

First and foremost, engaging in regular weight-bearing and resistance exercises is critical for strengthening bones. Activities like walking, dancing, and using weight machines can enhance bone density and improve balance, thereby reducing the risk of falls. Additionally, incorporating flexibility and balance exercises, such as yoga or tai chi, can further support stability and coordination. It is essential for postmenopausal women to consult with healthcare professionals to design an exercise program tailored to their individual capabilities and health conditions, ensuring safety while maximizing the benefits.

Nutrition plays a crucial role in osteoporosis management. A balanced diet rich in calcium and vitamin D is vital for bone health. Postmenopausal women should aim to include dairy products, leafy greens, and fortified foods in their diets to meet their calcium needs. Simultaneously, vitamin D can be obtained through sunlight exposure and fortified foods, or supplements if required. Adequate protein intake is also important, as it helps maintain muscle mass and bone strength. Women should work with dietitians to develop personalized meal plans that cater to their nutritional needs while considering any dietary restrictions.

In addition to lifestyle and dietary adjustments, medication management is a key element in controlling osteoporosis. There are various medications available, including bisphosphonates, hormone therapy, and newer agents like monoclonal antibodies. Each option has its benefits and risks, so it is crucial for patients to engage in open discussions with their healthcare providers to determine the most suitable treatment plan based on their specific medical history and risk factors. Adhering to prescribed medication regimens is fundamental to achieving optimal outcomes in bone health.

Finally, regular screening and monitoring for osteoporosis should not be overlooked. Women who are postmenopausal should discuss bone density testing with their healthcare providers to assess their risk for fractures and to establish a baseline for future evaluations. Regular follow-ups can help track the effectiveness of the chosen management strategies, allowing for timely adjustments as necessary. Early detection and proactive management can significantly reduce the chances of serious complications related to osteoporosis, ensuring that postmenopausal women can lead active and fulfilling lives.

Chapter 3: Pediatric Osteoporosis

Causes of Osteoporosis in Children

Osteoporosis in children, while less common than in adults, can have significant implications for lifelong bone health. Understanding the causes of pediatric osteoporosis is crucial for effective prevention and management.

One of the primary factors contributing to osteoporosis in children is genetic predisposition. Children with a family history of osteoporosis or related conditions may be at a higher risk, as genetics play a vital role in bone density and overall skeletal health. Genetic disorders such as osteogenesis imperfecta can also directly impact bone strength, leading to increased fragility and a higher likelihood of fractures.

Nutritional deficiencies are another critical factor affecting bone health in children. Calcium and vitamin D are essential for bone development and maintenance. A lack of these nutrients can hinder the body's ability to form new bone and repair existing tissue. Many children do not consume adequate amounts of dairy products or fortified foods, leading to insufficient calcium intake. Similarly, limited sunlight exposure can result in low vitamin D levels, further exacerbating the risk of developing osteoporosis. It is essential for parents and caregivers to ensure that children receive a balanced diet rich in these nutrients to support optimal bone growth.

Physical activity is vital for maintaining bone density, and a sedentary lifestyle can be a significant cause of osteoporosis in children. Weight-bearing exercises, such as running, jumping, and dancing, stimulate bone formation and increase bone strength. However, many children today are less active due to increased screen time and a lack of outdoor play. This decline in physical activity can lead to decreased bone mass during the critical years of growth. Encouraging regular exercise and active play can help mitigate this risk and promote healthier bones from a young age.

Hormonal factors also play a significant role in the development of osteoporosis in children. Conditions that disrupt normal hormonal balance, such as hyperthyroidism or certain endocrine disorders, can negatively affect bone health. Additionally, premature onset of puberty or delayed puberty can influence bone density, as the timing of hormonal changes impacts peak bone mass achievement. It is essential to monitor children's growth and development closely, as any significant deviations may warrant further evaluation by a healthcare provider.

Lastly, certain medical conditions and medications can contribute to the development of osteoporosis in children. Chronic diseases such as cystic fibrosis, rheumatoid arthritis, or diabetes may affect nutrient absorption and overall health, leading to weaker bones. Furthermore, some medications, particularly corticosteroids, can have detrimental effects on bone density. Parents and healthcare providers must work together to manage these conditions effectively while considering the implications for bone health. Early identification and intervention can help reduce the risk of osteoporosis and promote stronger, healthier bones in children.

Symptoms and Diagnosis in Pediatric Patients

Pediatric osteoporosis is a condition that, while less commonly discussed than its adult counterpart, poses significant health risks to children and adolescents. Recognizing the symptoms of osteoporosis in younger patients is crucial for timely intervention and management. Common signs may include recurrent fractures that occur from minimal trauma, as well as bone pain or tenderness. Children may also experience growth delays or have difficulty participating in physical activities due to weakness or fatigue. Parents should be vigilant about any unusual behaviors or complaints of pain that could indicate underlying bone health issues.

Diagnosis of osteoporosis in pediatric patients involves a combination of clinical evaluation and diagnostic testing. A thorough medical history is essential, including any family history of osteoporosis, nutritional habits, and physical activity levels. Physicians may conduct a physical examination and may inquire about dietary intake, particularly calcium and vitamin D, as these nutrients play a critical role in bone health. If osteoporosis is suspected, a dual-energy X-ray absorptiometry (DEXA) scan is often recommended to assess bone mineral density and help determine the risk of fractures.

In addition to imaging studies, blood tests may be utilized to rule out other conditions that could contribute to bone health issues, such as hormonal imbalances or metabolic disorders. These tests can measure levels of calcium, phosphorus, and vitamin D, as well as markers of bone turnover. Understanding the underlying causes of osteoporosis in children is essential, as pediatric osteoporosis can be secondary to other conditions, such as chronic diseases or prolonged use of certain medications, which can affect bone density negatively.

The approach to managing pediatric osteoporosis must be comprehensive and tailored to the individual needs of the child. This often includes nutritional counseling to ensure adequate intake of calcium and vitamin D, alongside recommendations for safe physical activity that promotes bone strength. In some cases, medications may be necessary, particularly if the child is at high risk for fractures. Ongoing monitoring and follow-up assessments are important to evaluate the effectiveness of the treatment plan and make adjustments as needed.

Education is key for both patients and families in managing pediatric osteoporosis. Parents should be informed about the importance of bone health and the factors that contribute to maintaining strong bones, such as proper nutrition, regular exercise, and avoiding smoking or excessive alcohol consumption. By fostering a supportive environment and encouraging healthy lifestyle choices, families can play a crucial role in enhancing their child's bone health and reducing the risk of future fractures. Awareness and proactive management can lead to better outcomes for children affected by osteoporosis.

Treatment Options and Lifestyle Adjustments

Treatment options for osteoporosis typically involve a combination of medication and lifestyle adjustments to strengthen bones and reduce the risk of fractures. Medications such as bisphosphonates, hormone replacement therapy, and newer agents like monoclonal antibodies play a crucial role in slowing bone loss and promoting bone density. Patients should engage in discussions with their healthcare providers to determine the most suitable medication based on individual health profiles, including age, gender, and the presence of other medical conditions. Regular follow-ups and monitoring are essential to assess the effectiveness of the chosen treatment and adjust it as necessary.

Lifestyle adjustments significantly complement medical treatments and can enhance overall bone health. Nutrition plays a vital role in managing osteoporosis; a diet rich in calcium and vitamin D is foundational for bone strength. Patients should focus on consuming dairy products, leafy greens, fatty fish, and fortified foods. Supplements may also be recommended when dietary intake is insufficient. Additionally, it is important to stay hydrated and limit excessive caffeine and alcohol consumption, as these can negatively impact bone density.

Physical activity is another cornerstone of osteoporosis management. Engaging in weight-bearing exercises, such as walking, jogging, or dancing, helps to stimulate bone formation and improve balance, thereby reducing the risk of falls and fractures. Strength training exercises can also be beneficial, as they help build muscle mass, which supports and protects the bones. For those with advanced osteoporosis or a history of fractures, low-impact exercises such as swimming or cycling may be advisable. Consulting with a physical therapist can help design an appropriate exercise regimen tailored to individual capabilities.

Screening and diagnosis of osteoporosis are crucial for early intervention and effective management. Patients, particularly postmenopausal women and men over 70, should undergo regular bone density tests to assess their bone health. These tests can identify individuals at high risk for fractures, allowing for timely treatment. Awareness of personal risk factors, such as family history, previous fractures, and lifestyle habits, can inform the need for screening and facilitate proactive measures.

Preventing osteoporosis should begin early in life, with an emphasis on building strong bones during childhood and adolescence. Ensuring adequate intake of nutrients, engaging in regular physical activity, and avoiding smoking can establish a strong foundation for bone health. Education about osteoporosis and its risk factors can empower patients and their families to adopt healthier lifestyles. By integrating effective treatment options with proactive lifestyle choices, individuals can significantly improve their bone health and reduce the risk of osteoporotic fractures throughout their lives.

Key Nutrients for Bone Health

Bone health is significantly influenced by key nutrients that play vital roles in bone formation, maintenance, and overall strength. Understanding these nutrients is essential for patients managing osteoporosis, as they provide a foundation for both prevention and treatment strategies. The primary nutrients critical for bone health include calcium, vitamin D, magnesium, and vitamin K, each contributing uniquely to skeletal integrity and resilience.

Calcium is the most abundant mineral in the body and a crucial component of bone tissue. It is essential for developing and maintaining strong bones, especially during the formative years in childhood and adolescence, as well as during postmenopausal years when bone density can decline. Adults should aim for a daily intake of 1,000 to 1,200 milligrams of calcium, depending on age and gender. Dairy products, leafy greens, and fortified foods are excellent sources of calcium. For those who struggle to meet their calcium needs through diet alone, supplements may be a necessary option, but should be discussed with a healthcare provider to ensure proper dosage and avoid potential side effects.

Vitamin D is another critical nutrient for bone health, as it enhances calcium absorption in the gut and helps regulate calcium levels in the blood. Without adequate vitamin D, bones can become thin, brittle, or misshapen. The body produces vitamin D through exposure to sunlight, but many individuals, especially those living in regions with limited sunlight or those who spend much time indoors, may require additional sources. Foods such as fatty fish, egg yolks, and fortified products can provide vitamin D, but supplementation may be necessary for those at risk of deficiency. Regular screening for vitamin D levels can also guide necessary interventions.

Magnesium plays a lesser-known yet significant role in bone health. It is involved in converting vitamin D into its active form, which is crucial for calcium absorption. Additionally, magnesium contributes to the structural development of bones and helps regulate calcium levels. Foods rich in magnesium include nuts, seeds, whole grains, and leafy green vegetables. Maintaining adequate magnesium levels can help prevent osteoporosis and support overall bone density. Patients should be aware of the interplay between magnesium and other nutrients, as an imbalance can affect bone health.

Vitamin K is essential for the synthesis of proteins involved in bone metabolism. It helps bind calcium to the bone matrix, thereby enhancing bone mineralization and reducing the risk of fractures. Leafy green vegetables, such as kale and spinach, as well as fermented foods, are rich sources of vitamin K. As with other nutrients, ensuring sufficient intake of vitamin K can be particularly important for individuals with osteoporosis. Patients should consider their dietary intake and consult with healthcare professionals to develop a balanced approach that incorporates all key nutrients necessary for optimal bone health. By prioritizing these essential nutrients, patients can take proactive steps toward managing osteoporosis effectively.

Dietary Sources of Calcium and Vitamin D

Calcium and vitamin D are critical nutrients for maintaining bone health, particularly for individuals at risk of osteoporosis. Adequate calcium intake is essential for the development and maintenance of strong bones. Dietary sources of calcium include dairy products such as milk, cheese, and yogurt, which are rich in this vital mineral. For those who are lactose intolerant or prefer non-dairy options, fortified plant-based milk alternatives, leafy green vegetables like kale and broccoli, and fortified foods such as cereals and orange juice can provide significant amounts of calcium. Understanding how to incorporate these foods into daily meals can help meet the recommended dietary allowances and support bone density.

Vitamin D plays a crucial role in calcium absorption and bone metabolism. The body can produce vitamin D when exposed to sunlight, but dietary sources are also important, especially for individuals who may have limited sun exposure. Fatty fish such as salmon, mackerel, and sardines are excellent natural sources of vitamin D. Additionally, fortified foods, including certain dairy products, cereals, and even some types of bread, can help boost vitamin D intake. For individuals who struggle to obtain enough vitamin D through diet and sunlight, supplements are a viable option and should be discussed with a healthcare provider to determine the appropriate dosage.

In pediatric populations, ensuring adequate intake of calcium and vitamin D is vital for optimal bone growth and development. During childhood and adolescence, the body builds the majority of bone mass, making good nutrition crucial during these formative years. Dairy products, fortified foods, and a balanced diet rich in fruits and vegetables can support healthy bone development. Encouraging children to engage in physical activities and outdoor play can also enhance vitamin D synthesis and promote strong bones.

Postmenopausal women face specific challenges related to bone health due to hormonal changes that affect bone density. As estrogen levels decline, the risk of osteoporosis increases, making adequate calcium and vitamin D intake even more important. Women should focus on incorporating calcium-rich foods into their diets while also ensuring they have sufficient vitamin D to facilitate calcium absorption. Regular screenings and discussions with healthcare providers about dietary needs can play a significant role in preventing osteoporosis-related fractures.

In older adults and individuals with chronic diseases, maintaining adequate levels of calcium and vitamin D is essential to prevent the progression of osteoporosis. Nutritional counseling can help tailor dietary plans that accommodate specific health conditions while ensuring bone health is prioritized. Rehabilitation programs for osteoporotic fractures often emphasize the importance of nutrition in recovery, reinforcing that proper dietary habits can enhance healing and improve overall bone strength. By prioritizing these nutrients, individuals can take proactive steps toward managing their bone health and reducing the risk of osteoporosis-related complications.

Nutritional Strategies for Osteoporosis Management

Nutritional strategies play a crucial role in managing osteoporosis and promoting bone health. Essential nutrients such as calcium and vitamin D are foundational in maintaining bone density and preventing fractures. Calcium is vital for bone formation, while vitamin D enhances calcium absorption in the intestines. For adults, particularly postmenopausal women who are at higher risk of osteoporosis, it is recommended to consume adequate amounts of calcium ranging from 1,200 mg per day. Foods rich in calcium include dairy products, leafy green vegetables, and fortified foods. Vitamin D can be obtained from fatty fish, fortified dairy products, and sunlight exposure, which is essential for overall bone health.

In addition to calcium and vitamin D, other nutrients significantly contribute to bone strength. Magnesium, potassium, and vitamins K and C are essential for optimal bone health. Magnesium aids in converting vitamin D into its active form and is found in whole grains, nuts, and seeds. Vitamin K, which is crucial for bone mineralization, can be found in green leafy vegetables. Vitamin C is important for collagen synthesis, a key component of bone structure, and is abundant in fruits and vegetables. Ensuring a well-rounded diet that includes these nutrients can help reinforce bone integrity and reduce the risk of osteoporosis-related fractures.

For individuals with osteoporosis or at risk, it is important to limit certain dietary components that may negatively affect bone health. High sodium intake can lead to increased calcium excretion through urine, potentially weakening bones over time. Processed foods, which are often high in sodium, should be consumed in moderation. Additionally, excessive caffeine consumption may interfere with calcium absorption and bone health. It is advisable for individuals to limit their caffeine intake to no more than 2-3 cups of coffee or its equivalent per day. Alcohol should also be consumed in moderation, as heavy drinking can lead to bone loss and increase the risk of falls and fractures.

Hydration is another often-overlooked aspect of bone health. Staying well-hydrated is essential for overall health, including bone integrity. Dehydration can lead to muscle weakness and increase the risk of falls, which is a significant concern for individuals with osteoporosis. Drinking adequate amounts of water throughout the day, along with consuming hydrating foods such as fruits and vegetables, can support both bone health and overall well-being. Patients should aim for at least eight glasses of water daily, adjusting based on individual needs and activity levels.

Finally, combining nutritional strategies with appropriate physical activity enhances bone health. Weight-bearing and resistance exercises help stimulate bone formation and improve balance, reducing the risk of falls. Patients should consult with healthcare providers to develop a tailored exercise plan that complements their nutritional strategies. By integrating a balanced diet rich in bone-supporting nutrients, limiting harmful substances, and engaging in regular physical activity, individuals can significantly improve their osteoporosis management and overall quality of life.

Chapter 5: Osteoporosis Medications and Treatments

Overview of Osteoporosis Medications

Osteoporosis medications are essential tools in managing this condition, which weakens bones and increases the risk of fractures. These medications work by either slowing down bone loss, enhancing bone formation, or both. The primary categories of osteoporosis medications include bisphosphonates, hormone-related therapies, and newer agents such as monoclonal antibodies. Understanding how these medications function and their potential benefits and side effects is crucial for patients seeking to strengthen their bones and minimize fracture risk.

Bisphosphonates are among the most commonly prescribed osteoporosis medications. They inhibit the activity of osteoclasts, the cells responsible for bone resorption, leading to a net gain in bone density. Medications like alendronate, risedronate, and zoledronic acid belong to this class. They are typically administered either orally or intravenously and can significantly reduce the risk of vertebral and hip fractures. However, patients should be aware of potential side effects, which may include gastrointestinal issues and, in rare cases, osteonecrosis of the jaw.

Hormone replacement therapy (HRT) is another option, particularly for postmenopausal women. Estrogen plays a vital role in maintaining bone density, and its decline after menopause can lead to rapid bone loss. HRT can help mitigate these effects by replenishing estrogen levels. While effective in reducing fracture risk, HRT is not suitable for everyone due to potential risks, such as cardiovascular disease and certain cancers. Therefore, it is essential for patients to discuss their medical history and risk factors with their healthcare provider before considering this treatment.

Recent advancements have led to the development of monoclonal antibodies like denosumab, which target specific pathways in bone metabolism. Denosumab works by inhibiting RANKL, a protein that promotes the formation and activity of osteoclasts. This medication is administered via subcutaneous injection and has demonstrated effectiveness in increasing bone density and reducing fracture risk. Additionally, new anabolic agents, such as teriparatide, stimulate bone formation by mimicking parathyroid hormone. These treatments provide exciting alternatives for patients, especially those with more severe osteoporosis or those who cannot tolerate traditional therapies.

It's important for patients to engage in a comprehensive care plan that includes medication management alongside lifestyle modifications. Factors such as nutrition, exercise, and fall prevention play crucial roles in managing osteoporosis effectively. Patients should also be proactive in discussing their treatment options with healthcare professionals, ensuring they understand the benefits and risks of each medication. Regular monitoring and follow-up appointments are essential to assess the effectiveness of the treatment and make necessary adjustments, ultimately leading to stronger bones and improved quality of life.

Benefits and Risks of Common Treatments

Common treatments for osteoporosis, including medications, lifestyle changes, and nutritional interventions, come with a range of benefits and risks that patients should carefully consider. Medications such as bisphosphonates, denosumab, and hormone replacement therapy can effectively increase bone density and reduce the risk of fractures. These treatments can significantly improve quality of life, especially for postmenopausal women and older adults who are at higher risk. However, patients must also be aware of potential side effects, which can include gastrointestinal issues, musculoskeletal pain, and, in rare cases, more severe complications like osteonecrosis of the jaw or atypical femur fractures.

Lifestyle changes, such as incorporating weight-bearing exercises and engaging in fall prevention strategies, are also cornerstone treatments for osteoporosis. Regular exercise can enhance muscle strength, balance, and coordination, reducing the likelihood of falls and subsequent fractures. Furthermore, participating in physical activity promotes overall health and well-being. However, patients need to approach exercise cautiously, particularly if they have existing fractures or severe bone loss, as certain high-impact activities could pose a risk of injury.

Nutritional interventions play an essential role in managing osteoporosis. A diet rich in calcium and vitamin D is crucial for bone health, as these nutrients are fundamental for bone formation and maintenance. Foods such as dairy products, leafy greens, and fortified foods can help meet these dietary needs. Nevertheless, patients should be cautious about excessive supplementation, which can lead to kidney stones or cardiovascular issues. Consulting with a healthcare provider or a registered dietitian can ensure that nutritional strategies are both safe and effective.

When considering osteoporosis treatments, screening and early diagnosis are paramount. Regular bone density tests can help identify individuals at risk and facilitate timely intervention. Early treatment can prevent the progression of osteoporosis and reduce the incidence of fractures. However, patients may be apprehensive about the testing process and the potential for false positives or negatives. It is important to have open discussions with healthcare providers about the implications of test results and the most appropriate follow-up actions.

Finally, patients with osteoporosis must weigh the benefits of treatment against their personal health profiles and risk factors. Chronic diseases, such as diabetes or rheumatoid arthritis, can influence treatment choices and outcomes. Additionally, individual preferences and comfort levels regarding medications and lifestyle changes should be taken into account. Engaging in shared decision-making with healthcare providers can empower patients to take an active role in their osteoporosis management, enabling them to choose the most suitable treatment options while being mindful of the associated benefits and risks.

Emerging Therapies and Research

Emerging therapies and research in the field of osteoporosis are vital for improving patient outcomes and quality of life. Recent advancements focus on developing innovative treatments that target bone density and overall skeletal health. Among these, biologics such as monoclonal antibodies have garnered significant attention. These therapies work by inhibiting specific pathways that lead to bone resorption, thereby promoting the formation of new bone. For instance, denosumab has demonstrated effectiveness in reducing the risk of fractures in postmenopausal women, which is crucial given their higher susceptibility to osteoporosis. Continued clinical trials and studies are essential to determine the long-term effects and potential applications of these therapies across diverse patient populations.

Research into osteoporosis in pediatric populations is also making strides. Traditionally considered a condition primarily affecting older adults, osteoporosis can also manifest in children, particularly those with chronic illnesses or specific genetic predispositions. Emerging therapies in this area include the use of bisphosphonates and other medications that have shown promise in improving bone density in young patients. Additionally, studies are increasingly focusing on the role of nutrition and physical activity in bone health during childhood and adolescence. Understanding the implications of these factors can lead to more effective prevention strategies and treatment protocols tailored to younger patients.

Nutritional interventions remain a cornerstone of osteoporosis management, and ongoing research continues to explore the role of specific nutrients in bone health. Calcium and vitamin D have long been recognized for their importance, but emerging studies are examining the effects of additional micronutrients such as magnesium, zinc, and vitamin K. Furthermore, the relationship between dietary patterns and bone health is being investigated, with particular attention to the Mediterranean diet, which is rich in fruits, vegetables, whole grains, and healthy fats. These insights could pave the way for more personalized dietary recommendations that support bone health in various demographics, including postmenopausal women and men.

Exercise physiology is another promising area of research, with new findings highlighting the importance of weight-bearing and resistance training in maintaining and improving bone density. Emerging studies are investigating the optimal types, intensities, and durations of exercise that can yield the best outcomes for individuals with osteoporosis. Tailored exercise programs are being developed that consider the unique needs of different populations, including older adults and those recovering from osteoporotic fractures. This research not only emphasizes the role of physical activity in preventing bone loss but also illustrates how rehabilitation can be integrated into comprehensive osteoporosis management plans.

Screening and diagnosis of osteoporosis are evolving, with technology playing a crucial role in early detection and intervention. Research is focusing on the development of advanced imaging techniques and biomarkers that can identify individuals at risk more accurately. Additionally, studies are investigating the psychological and social factors that influence osteoporosis management, particularly in men and postmenopausal women. By understanding these dynamics, healthcare providers can develop more effective screening guidelines and personalized treatment plans that address both the physical and emotional aspects of living with osteoporosis. As these emerging therapies and research findings continue to unfold, they hold the potential to transform the landscape of osteoporosis management, providing hope and improved outcomes for patients.

Chapter 6: Osteoporosis and Exercise Physiology

Importance of Exercise for Bone Health

Exercise plays a crucial role in maintaining and enhancing bone health, particularly for individuals at risk of osteoporosis. Engaging in regular physical activity helps to stimulate bone formation and improve bone density, which is vital for reducing the risk of fractures and other complications associated with weakened bones. For patients with osteoporosis or those at risk, understanding the types and benefits of exercise can empower them to incorporate physical activity into their daily routines effectively.

Weight-bearing and resistance exercises are particularly beneficial for building and maintaining bone density. Weight-bearing activities, such as walking, jogging, or dancing, force the body to work against gravity, thus stimulating bone growth. Resistance training, which includes using weights or resistance bands, helps strengthen the muscles surrounding the bones, providing additional support and stability. These exercises not only enhance bone strength but also improve overall muscle function and balance, reducing the likelihood of falls and subsequent fractures.

For postmenopausal women, the importance of exercise cannot be overstated. After menopause, bone density decreases significantly due to a drop in estrogen levels, making exercise an essential component of osteoporosis management. Engaging in a consistent exercise program can help mitigate bone loss and improve overall health. Strength training has been shown to be particularly effective in promoting bone density in this demographic, making it a crucial focus for prevention strategies.

Children and adolescents are also at a critical stage for bone health. The foundation for strong bones is laid during these formative years, making physical activity essential for developing optimal bone mass. Pediatric osteoporosis can lead to long-term consequences if not addressed early. Encouraging children to participate in weight-bearing sports and activities helps them build strong bones, which can have lasting effects into adulthood. It is important for parents and caregivers to promote an active lifestyle from a young age to prevent osteoporosis later in life.

In addition to the physical benefits, exercise can also have a positive impact on mental health and well-being. Engaging in regular physical activity releases endorphins, which can help alleviate symptoms of anxiety and depression that may accompany a diagnosis of osteoporosis. Furthermore, exercise can foster social connections through group activities or classes, creating a supportive environment for individuals managing their condition. By recognizing the multifaceted benefits of exercise, patients can be motivated to make it an integral part of their osteoporosis management plan.

Types of Exercises Beneficial for Osteoporosis

When managing osteoporosis, understanding the types of exercises that can be beneficial is critical for maintaining bone health and overall well-being. Resistance training, also known as strength training, is particularly effective as it involves lifting weights or using resistance bands to enhance muscle strength and bone density. These exercises create stress on the bones, stimulating the bone-forming cells to produce new bone tissue. For patients with osteoporosis, it is essential to begin with lighter weights and gradually increase resistance under the guidance of a healthcare professional to ensure safety and effectiveness.

Weight-bearing exercises are another vital component in the exercise regimen for individuals with osteoporosis. These activities, which include walking, jogging, dancing, and climbing stairs, require the body to work against gravity. Such exercises encourage bone remodeling and can help maintain or even improve bone density. Patients should aim for at least 30 minutes of weight-bearing activity most days of the week, while also incorporating balance exercises to reduce the risk of falls and fractures.

Balance and flexibility exercises are crucial for individuals with osteoporosis, especially postmenopausal women who may experience increased risks due to hormonal changes. Activities such as yoga, tai chi, and simple stretching routines can enhance proprioception and coordination, reducing the likelihood of falls. These exercises not only improve stability but also promote relaxation and well-being, which are important for overall health management in osteoporosis.

Aquatic exercises present a low-impact option for osteoporosis patients, particularly those with joint pain or mobility issues. Water buoyancy reduces stress on the bones and joints while providing resistance to strengthen muscles. Swimming, water aerobics, and other water-based activities can be excellent choices for maintaining fitness without the risk of injury. Patients should ensure that any aquatic programs are designed to accommodate their specific needs and capabilities.

Finally, it is essential to approach exercise with a comprehensive plan that considers individual health status, level of physical fitness, and specific osteoporosis risks. Consultation with healthcare providers, physical therapists, or certified trainers specializing in osteoporosis can help tailor an exercise program that promotes bone health while minimizing the risk of injury. By integrating various types of exercises into their routine, individuals with osteoporosis can significantly enhance their quality of life and better manage their condition.

Creating an Exercise Plan

Creating an exercise plan tailored for individuals with osteoporosis is essential for strengthening bones and enhancing overall health. Exercise can play a pivotal role in preventing fractures and improving balance, which is particularly crucial for those at risk. When formulating an exercise plan, it is vital to consider the specific needs and limitations of the individual, including their age, gender, medical history, and current fitness level. Engaging with healthcare professionals, such as physical therapists or exercise physiologists, can provide valuable guidance in developing a safe and effective program.

A well-rounded exercise plan for osteoporosis should incorporate three main components: weight-bearing exercises, strength training, and balance activities. Weight-bearing exercises, such as walking, dancing, or low-impact aerobics, help stimulate bone formation by forcing the body to work against gravity. Strength training, using resistance bands or weights, builds muscle strength and can improve bone density. Additionally, balance exercises like tai chi or yoga enhance coordination and stability, reducing the risk of falls and subsequent fractures.

When creating an exercise plan, it is crucial to start slowly and gradually increase the intensity and duration of workouts. This approach allows the body to adapt, minimizing the risk of injury. Patients should aim for at least 30 minutes of physical activity most days of the week, though this can be broken into shorter sessions if necessary. Listening to one's body and adjusting the exercise routine according to how one feels on a given day is essential for long-term adherence and success.

Safety is paramount when exercising with osteoporosis. It is advisable to avoid high-impact activities, such as running or jumping, which could increase the risk of fractures. Additionally, exercises that require bending forward or twisting motions should be approached with caution, as they may strain the spine. Proper footwear and a safe exercise environment are equally important to prevent slips and falls. Regular check-ins with a healthcare provider can help ensure that the exercise plan remains appropriate as the individual's condition evolves.

Finally, incorporating nutritional elements into the exercise plan can further support bone health. Adequate calcium and vitamin D intake plays a critical role in bone density, and patients should consider how their diet complements their physical activity. Hydration is also essential to maintain energy levels during workouts. By combining a tailored exercise plan with a balanced diet, individuals can take significant steps toward managing their osteoporosis effectively, enhancing their overall quality of life and reducing the risk of fractures.

Chapter 7: Osteoporosis Screening and Diagnosis

Understanding Bone Density Tests

Bone density tests are essential tools in diagnosing and managing osteoporosis, providing valuable insights into an individual's bone health. These tests measure the amount of mineral content in bones, particularly calcium and phosphorus, which are crucial for maintaining bone strength. The results help healthcare providers assess the risk of fractures and determine the severity of bone loss. Understanding how these tests work, their different types, and what the results mean can empower patients to take proactive steps in managing their osteoporosis.

The most commonly used bone density test is the Dual-Energy X-ray Absorptiometry (DEXA) scan. This non-invasive procedure involves lying on a table while a machine passes over the body, measuring bone density at key sites such as the hip and spine. The DEXA scan is quick, typically taking only 10 to 30 minutes, and exposes patients to minimal radiation, making it a safe option for regular screening. For pediatric patients, specialized pediatric DEXA machines are available to ensure accurate assessments tailored to their growing bodies.

Bone density tests provide results in the form of T-scores and Z-scores. The T-score compares an individual's bone density to that of a healthy young adult, while the Z-score compares it to individuals of the same age and sex. A T-score of -1.0 or higher is considered normal, between -1.0 and -2.5 indicates low bone mass (osteopenia), and -2.5 or lower confirms osteoporosis. Understanding these scores is crucial for patients, as they inform treatment decisions and lifestyle changes aimed at improving bone health.

Regular bone density testing is particularly important for certain groups, including postmenopausal women, men over 70, and individuals with risk factors such as chronic diseases or a family history of osteoporosis. The National Osteoporosis Foundation recommends that women begin screening at age 65 and that men start at age 70. For those with risk factors, earlier testing may be warranted. By identifying low bone density early, patients can work with their healthcare providers to implement prevention strategies and treatments that can help mitigate further bone loss.

In addition to understanding the test results, patients should be aware of the importance of follow-up testing. Bone density can fluctuate over time due to various factors such as medication adherence, lifestyle changes, and overall health. Regular monitoring allows for timely adjustments in treatment plans, ensuring that patients are taking the most effective steps to strengthen their bones. By staying informed and engaged in their care, patients can play an active role in managing osteoporosis and maintaining their quality of life.

Who Should Be Screened?

Screening for osteoporosis is crucial for identifying individuals at risk of developing the disease and preventing serious complications such as fractures. Generally, certain populations are more likely to benefit from screening due to their increased risk factors. Postmenopausal women are at the highest risk because the decrease in estrogen levels following menopause significantly accelerates bone loss. Therefore, women who are 65 years or older, or those under 65 with additional risk factors such as a family history of osteoporosis, previous fractures, or long-term use of corticosteroids, should be screened regularly.

Additionally, men are often overlooked in discussions about osteoporosis, but they also face significant risks. While osteoporosis is more common in women, men can experience bone density loss, particularly after the age of 70 or if they have risk factors such as low testosterone levels, chronic diseases, or a history of smoking and excessive alcohol consumption. Men with these characteristics should consider screening to assess their bone health and take proactive steps to maintain strong bones.

Pediatric osteoporosis, although less common, is an important concern that warrants attention. Children and adolescents can develop osteoporosis due to various factors such as genetic predispositions, medical conditions like cystic fibrosis or juvenile arthritis, or the use of certain medications. Screening in this population is particularly valuable for those who have experienced fractures with minimal trauma or who have conditions affecting bone health. Early identification can lead to interventions that support healthy bone development during critical growth periods.

Nutrition plays a vital role in bone health, and individuals with dietary deficiencies or eating disorders may be at risk of osteoporosis. Those with low calcium and vitamin D intake or conditions that affect nutrient absorption, such as celiac disease, should be evaluated for bone density. Screening can help identify individuals who may benefit from dietary modifications or supplements to enhance their bone health.

Lastly, individuals with chronic diseases that impact bone health, such as rheumatoid arthritis or chronic kidney disease, should also be screened for osteoporosis. These conditions often lead to changes in bone metabolism and can increase the risk of fractures. Regular screening can facilitate early diagnosis and management, allowing for tailored interventions that address both the underlying disease and the associated risk of osteoporosis. By identifying and screening at-risk individuals, healthcare providers can implement effective prevention and treatment strategies, ultimately reducing the incidence of osteoporotic fractures.

Interpreting Your Results

Interpreting your results after undergoing screening for osteoporosis is a crucial step in managing your bone health. The results of bone density tests, typically reported as T-scores and Z-scores, provide insight into your bone mineral density (BMD) compared to healthy individuals of the same age and sex. Understanding these scores is vital for determining your risk of fractures and guiding treatment options. A T-score of -1.0 or higher is considered normal, while scores between -1.0 and -2.5 indicate low bone density, or osteopenia. A score of -2.5 or lower signifies osteoporosis. Recognizing where you stand on this spectrum can empower you to take proactive measures in your treatment journey.

In the context of postmenopausal women, interpreting results becomes even more significant due to the accelerated bone loss that often occurs after menopause. Women in this demographic should pay close attention to their T-scores, as they are at a higher risk for developing osteoporosis. If your results indicate osteopenia or osteoporosis, it is essential to discuss with your healthcare provider the implications of these findings, including potential lifestyle changes and treatment options. Understanding the relationship between hormonal changes and bone density can motivate you to take steps that may help to mitigate further bone loss.

For pediatric patients, interpreting osteoporosis results requires a slightly different approach. In children, the focus is not only on BMD but also on growth patterns and bone development. Results should be evaluated in conjunction with clinical assessments to determine if the child is at risk for fractures. Pediatric osteoporosis may stem from various factors, including genetic conditions, nutritional deficiencies, or chronic diseases. Collaborating with a pediatrician or a specialist in pediatric bone health can help in deciphering the results and formulating a comprehensive management plan that addresses both bone health and overall growth.

Nutrition plays a pivotal role in bone health, and the interpretation of your results can guide dietary choices. If your bone density results indicate low bone mass, it may be an indication that your diet lacks sufficient calcium and vitamin D, both essential for bone strength. Discussing your results with a nutritionist can help you design a meal plan that supports bone health. This can include incorporating foods rich in these nutrients or considering supplements if necessary. By understanding how your results correlate with your nutritional intake, you can take actionable steps towards strengthening your bones.

Lastly, understanding your results in the context of potential treatments and exercises is essential for effective osteoporosis management. If your bone density results indicate osteoporosis, your healthcare provider may recommend medications that can help to strengthen bones and reduce the risk of fractures. Additionally, interpreting your results can inform your exercise regimen. Weight-bearing and resistance exercises are particularly beneficial for building bone strength. Engaging in regular physical activity, tailored to your individual needs and abilities, can significantly improve your outcomes. By interpreting your results holistically, you can develop a personalized strategy that encompasses medication, nutrition, and exercise to promote optimal bone health.

Chapter 8: Osteoporosis in Men

Prevalence and Risk Factors in Men

The prevalence of osteoporosis in men, while lower than in women, is a significant concern due to its growing recognition as a major health issue. Research indicates that approximately one in four men over the age of 50 will experience an osteoporotic fracture in their lifetime. This statistic highlights the importance of awareness and early intervention, as men often remain undiagnosed and untreated compared to their female counterparts. The misconception that osteoporosis predominantly affects women can lead to a lack of screening and preventative measures in men, increasing their risk of fractures and associated complications.

Various risk factors contribute to the development of osteoporosis in men. Age is a primary factor, as bone density naturally decreases with advancing years. Additionally, low testosterone levels, which can occur due to aging or other medical conditions, significantly impact bone health. Lifestyle choices also play a crucial role; men who smoke, consume excessive alcohol, or lead a sedentary lifestyle are at higher risk. Furthermore, certain medical conditions, such as rheumatoid arthritis, chronic kidney disease, and gastrointestinal disorders, can hinder nutrient absorption and lead to decreased bone density.

Genetics also plays a significant role in determining an individual's risk for osteoporosis. A family history of osteoporosis or fractures can indicate a higher likelihood of developing the condition. Moreover, men with low body weight or those who have experienced significant weight loss are at an increased risk, as lower body mass can correlate with decreased bone density. Understanding these risk factors is essential for men to take proactive steps in maintaining their bone health.

Nutrition is another critical aspect in managing osteoporosis risk in men. A diet low in calcium and vitamin D can contribute to weakened bones. Men should aim to include calcium-rich foods such as dairy products, leafy greens, and fortified foods in their diets, alongside adequate vitamin D from sunlight exposure or supplements. Additionally, maintaining a balanced diet that supports overall health is vital, as malnutrition can exacerbate bone density loss.

Regular screening and early diagnosis are key in managing osteoporosis in men. Men over the age of 50, especially those with risk factors, should discuss bone density testing with their healthcare providers. Early detection allows for timely intervention, which may include lifestyle modifications, nutritional support, and medication when necessary. By addressing these factors and prioritizing bone health, men can significantly reduce their risk of osteoporosis and its associated fractures, leading to a healthier, more active life.

Symptoms and Diagnosis

Symptoms of osteoporosis can often be subtle and may go unnoticed until a fracture occurs. Many patients may not experience any symptoms in the early stages of bone loss, which is why osteoporosis is often referred to as a "silent disease." It is important to understand that the first indication of osteoporosis for many individuals, especially postmenopausal women, is typically a fracture resulting from a low-impact event, such as a fall from standing height. Common sites for these fractures include the hip, wrist, and spine. As osteoporosis progresses, some patients may experience other symptoms, such as back pain, loss of height, or a stooped posture, which can signal vertebral fractures.

Diagnosis of osteoporosis usually begins with a thorough medical history and physical examination. Healthcare providers will assess risk factors, including age, sex, family history, previous fractures, and lifestyle choices such as diet and exercise. This information helps to create a comprehensive picture of an individual's bone health. The most definitive method for diagnosing osteoporosis is through a Dual-energy X-ray Absorptiometry (DEXA) scan. This specialized imaging test measures bone mineral density (BMD) and compares it to established norms, providing a T-score that indicates whether an individual has normal bone density, low bone mass, or osteoporosis.

For postmenopausal women, the importance of early detection cannot be overstated. This demographic is at a higher risk for developing osteoporosis due to hormonal changes that occur during menopause. Therefore, it is recommended that women over the age of 65, or those with risk factors, undergo routine screening for osteoporosis. However, pediatric osteoporosis, although less common, should not be overlooked. Diagnosis in younger populations may involve assessing underlying conditions, family history, and lifestyle factors, as well as conducting appropriate imaging studies.

In addition to DEXA scans, other diagnostic tools may be utilized to evaluate bone health and assess the risk of fractures. These can include quantitative computed tomography (QCT) and various blood tests to measure calcium, vitamin D, and other markers of bone metabolism. It is essential for patients to engage in discussions with their healthcare providers about their specific risk factors and the appropriate timing for screening, particularly if they have experienced fractures or have chronic diseases that may impact bone density.

Recognizing the symptoms and understanding the diagnostic process for osteoporosis empowers patients to take control of their bone health. By being proactive and seeking regular assessments, individuals can identify low bone density early and implement strategies to strengthen their bones. This is particularly crucial for populations at risk, such as postmenopausal women and older adults, as timely diagnosis can lead to effective management and prevention of fractures, ultimately improving quality of life and mobility.

Treatment and Management Strategies

Treatment and management strategies for osteoporosis are essential to maintaining bone health and preventing fractures, particularly for specific populations such as postmenopausal women, children, and men. A multifaceted approach that includes medication, nutrition, exercise, and regular screening can significantly improve outcomes for individuals with osteoporosis. Understanding these strategies can empower patients and caregivers to take proactive steps in managing this condition.

Medications play a crucial role in the treatment of osteoporosis. Bisphosphonates, such as alendronate and risedronate, are commonly prescribed to reduce bone loss and lower the risk of fractures. Other options include denosumab, a monoclonal antibody that inhibits bone resorption, and teriparatide, a form of parathyroid hormone that promotes new bone formation. In some cases, hormone replacement therapy may be considered for postmenopausal women to help maintain bone density. Patients should have open discussions with their healthcare providers to determine the most appropriate medication based on individual risk factors and health status.

Nutrition is another cornerstone of osteoporosis management. Adequate intake of calcium and vitamin D is vital for maintaining strong bones. Foods rich in calcium, such as dairy products, leafy greens, and fortified foods, should be incorporated into daily meals. Vitamin D, which can be obtained from sunlight exposure and dietary sources, is essential for calcium absorption. In some cases, supplements may be recommended to ensure that individuals meet their nutritional needs. A well-balanced diet that includes a variety of nutrients contributes to overall bone health and can aid in the management of osteoporosis.

Exercise physiology plays a significant role in strengthening bones and preventing fractures. Weight-bearing and resistance exercises are particularly beneficial for individuals with osteoporosis. Activities such as walking, dancing, and strength training help stimulate bone formation and improve muscle strength, balance, and coordination. Patients should work with healthcare professionals to develop a personalized exercise program that is safe and effective, taking into consideration their current fitness level and any existing medical conditions. Regular physical activity not only supports bone health but also enhances overall well-being.

Regular screening and diagnosis are vital components of osteoporosis management, especially for high-risk groups. Bone density tests, like dual-energy X-ray absorptiometry (DXA), can identify low bone mass and predict fracture risk. Early detection allows for timely intervention, which can significantly reduce the likelihood of osteoporotic fractures. For patients with chronic diseases, additional assessments may be necessary to understand how their condition affects bone health. By prioritizing screenings and maintaining open communication with healthcare providers, patients can stay informed and actively participate in their osteoporosis management strategies.

Chapter 9: Osteoporosis Prevention Strategies

Lifestyle Changes for Prevention

Lifestyle changes play a crucial role in the prevention of osteoporosis and the maintenance of strong bones. Individuals at risk, particularly postmenopausal women, children, and men, can significantly benefit from implementing specific strategies that promote bone health. These changes encompass various aspects of daily life, including dietary modifications, physical activity, and the avoidance of harmful habits. By adopting a proactive approach to lifestyle, patients can enhance their overall well-being and reduce the likelihood of developing osteoporosis or experiencing fractures.

Nutrition is foundational for bone health. A diet rich in calcium and vitamin D is essential for building and maintaining bone density. Calcium sources include dairy products, leafy green vegetables, and fortified foods, while vitamin D can be obtained through sunlight exposure and supplements. Additionally, a diet that includes plenty of fruits and vegetables provides important antioxidants and phytochemicals that can help protect bone health. It is also advisable to limit the intake of sodium and caffeine, as excessive consumption can lead to calcium loss, further jeopardizing bone integrity.

Regular exercise is another critical component of osteoporosis prevention. Weight-bearing and resistance exercises are particularly effective in promoting bone strength. Activities such as walking, jogging, dancing, and strength training stimulate bone formation and help maintain bone density. For children and adolescents, engaging in sports and physical activities fosters a foundation for strong bones that can last into adulthood. For older adults, exercises that improve balance and coordination, such as tai chi or yoga, can help prevent falls, reducing the risk of fractures.

Lifestyle choices also play a significant role in bone health. Smoking has been linked to decreased bone density, as it affects the body's ability to absorb calcium and impairs estrogen production in women. Additionally, excessive alcohol consumption can interfere with calcium balance and hormone levels, further increasing the risk of osteoporosis. Therefore, quitting smoking and moderating alcohol intake are crucial steps patients can take to protect their bones. These changes not only benefit bone health but also enhance overall physical health and longevity.

Finally, regular screening and monitoring for osteoporosis are essential, especially for those at higher risk. Early diagnosis can lead to timely interventions, including lifestyle modifications and medical treatments when necessary. Patients should engage in open discussions with healthcare providers about their bone health, risk factors, and appropriate screening schedules. By taking proactive steps and making informed lifestyle choices, individuals can significantly reduce their risk of osteoporosis and its associated complications, ensuring a healthier and more active life.

Importance of Early Intervention

Early intervention in osteoporosis is crucial for effectively managing the condition and minimizing its long-term impact on bone health.

Osteoporosis is often a silent disease, with many individuals unaware of their weakened bone density until they experience a fracture. By recognizing the importance of early intervention, patients can take proactive steps to strengthen their bones and reduce the risk of fractures. This includes understanding the risk factors associated with osteoporosis, such as age, gender, family history, and lifestyle choices, which are particularly relevant for postmenopausal women and men.

One of the primary benefits of early intervention is the opportunity to implement preventive strategies before significant bone loss occurs. For both pediatric and adult patients, early diagnosis through screening can identify those at higher risk for osteoporosis. For instance, children with conditions that affect bone growth can benefit from early nutritional guidance and exercise regimens designed to support bone health. In postmenopausal women, timely interventions can help mitigate the rapid decline in bone density that often accompanies hormonal changes.

Nutrition plays a vital role in maintaining bone health, and early intervention provides the chance to educate patients on dietary choices that support strong bones. Adequate calcium and vitamin D intake are essential for bone development and maintenance. By addressing nutritional needs early on, patients can establish healthy eating habits that promote bone density. This is particularly important for individuals with osteoporosis or those at risk, as their dietary requirements may differ significantly from the general population.

Medication options for osteoporosis have advanced significantly, and early intervention allows for a tailored approach to treatment. Patients diagnosed with osteoporosis can work closely with their healthcare providers to determine the most appropriate medication based on their unique medical history and lifestyle. Early treatment can not only prevent further bone loss but can also improve overall bone quality, thereby reducing the risk of osteoporotic fractures. The sooner medication is initiated, the greater the potential for positive outcomes in bone health.

Lastly, integrating exercise into an osteoporosis management plan is vital for enhancing bone strength and overall physical well-being. Early intervention encourages patients to adopt a regular exercise routine that includes weight-bearing and resistance exercises, which are proven to stimulate bone formation. For those who have already experienced fractures, rehabilitation programs can be designed to accommodate their needs while promoting safe movement and strength building. By addressing osteoporosis through early intervention, patients can significantly improve their quality of life and reduce the risk of future complications associated with the disease.

Community Resources and Support

Community resources and support play a crucial role in managing osteoporosis and improving the quality of life for those affected by the condition. Patients can benefit from a variety of local and national organizations that provide information, advocacy, and resources tailored to their specific needs. These resources often include educational materials, workshops, and seminars aimed at increasing awareness about osteoporosis, its risk factors, and the importance of prevention and treatment strategies. Engaging with these organizations can empower patients to take charge of their health and connect with others facing similar challenges.

For postmenopausal women, specialized support groups and programs are available that focus on osteoporosis education and management. These groups often offer discussions led by healthcare professionals who can provide insights into the unique risks associated with menopause and bone health. Additionally, women can share personal experiences and coping strategies, fostering a sense of community and understanding. This peer support can be invaluable in navigating the emotional and physical challenges of living with osteoporosis.

Pediatric osteoporosis presents unique challenges, and families can find support through resources specifically designed for children and adolescents. Organizations dedicated to childhood bone health often offer guidance on nutrition, physical activity, and medication management tailored to younger patients. Educational materials for parents and caregivers can help them understand the importance of early diagnosis and intervention, ensuring that children receive the necessary care to optimize their bone health as they grow.

Nutrition plays a pivotal role in bone health, and community resources can assist patients in making informed dietary choices. Local health departments, nutritionists, and dietitians may offer workshops that focus on calcium and vitamin D intake, as well as other nutrients essential for bone strength. Additionally, cooking classes and meal planning sessions can help patients incorporate bone-healthy foods into their diets, making it easier to adhere to dietary recommendations. This support is particularly beneficial for those who may feel overwhelmed by the dietary changes needed to manage their osteoporosis effectively.

Finally, exercise physiology resources can guide patients in developing safe and effective exercise routines to strengthen bones and improve overall physical health. Community centers or local gyms may offer classes specifically designed for individuals with osteoporosis, focusing on low-impact activities that enhance strength, balance, and coordination. These classes not only promote physical health but also provide social interaction, reducing feelings of isolation. By taking advantage of these community resources, patients can find the support they need to manage osteoporosis proactively and improve their overall well-being.

Chapter 10: Osteoporosis and Chronic Diseases

Connection Between Chronic Diseases and Osteoporosis

Chronic diseases can significantly impact bone health, particularly in individuals with osteoporosis. The relationship between chronic diseases and osteoporosis is complex, as both conditions can exacerbate one another. For instance, conditions such as diabetes, rheumatoid arthritis, and chronic kidney disease can lead to a higher risk of bone density loss.

In patients with osteoporosis, the presence of these chronic diseases may contribute to a greater likelihood of fractures and complicate the healing process. Understanding this connection is vital for patients managing osteoporosis and other health issues.

Diabetes is one of the most common chronic diseases that can negatively affect bone health. Research indicates that both type 1 and type 2 diabetes are associated with lower bone mineral density. In individuals with type 1 diabetes, the lack of insulin can lead to decreased bone formation, while type 2 diabetes often involves insulin resistance, which can affect bone remodeling and strength. Patients with diabetes must be particularly vigilant about their bone health and may require tailored osteoporosis management strategies that consider their diabetic condition.

Rheumatoid arthritis (RA) presents another challenge for patients with osteoporosis. This autoimmune disease not only causes inflammation in the joints but can also lead to increased bone resorption, thereby accelerating bone loss. The use of corticosteroids to manage RA further amplifies this risk, as these medications are known to interfere with calcium absorption and inhibit bone formation. Patients with RA must engage in proactive osteoporosis management, including regular screening and potentially modifying their treatment regimens to mitigate bone loss.

Chronic kidney disease (CKD) is another condition that can adversely affect bone health. As kidney function declines, the body's ability to maintain calcium and phosphate balance is disrupted, leading to mineral and bone disorders. Patients with CKD often experience secondary hyperparathyroidism, which can cause further bone density loss. It is essential for patients with osteoporosis and CKD to work closely with their healthcare providers to monitor their bone health and adjust their treatment plans accordingly.

Patients with osteoporosis should also be aware of how lifestyle factors related to chronic diseases can impact their bone health. For example, sedentary behavior common in individuals with chronic illnesses can lead to further bone density loss. Engaging in weight-bearing exercises and maintaining a balanced diet rich in calcium and vitamin D are essential strategies for all patients, particularly those with both osteoporosis and chronic diseases. By understanding the interplay between these conditions, patients can take proactive steps to protect their bone health and improve their overall well-being.

Managing Osteoporosis with Coexisting Conditions

Managing osteoporosis becomes increasingly complex when coexisting conditions are present. These conditions can include chronic diseases such as diabetes, rheumatoid arthritis, and cardiovascular diseases, which may influence both the management of osteoporosis and the overall health of the patient. When dealing with osteoporosis, it is crucial to consider how these coexisting conditions may affect bone health and the effectiveness of treatment options. Understanding the interplay between osteoporosis and other health issues can lead to more tailored and effective management strategies.

In postmenopausal women, osteoporosis is often accompanied by conditions such as hypertension or hyperlipidemia. The medications used to manage these conditions may have side effects that impact bone density. For instance, certain antihypertensive medications can influence calcium metabolism or create a risk for falls, which can lead to fractures. Therefore, it is vital for patients to communicate openly with their healthcare providers about all medications they are taking, ensuring that both osteoporosis and coexisting conditions are addressed in a comprehensive manner.

In pediatric populations, the challenges of managing osteoporosis alongside other health issues, such as cystic fibrosis or juvenile idiopathic arthritis, can be particularly pronounced. Medications used to manage these conditions can affect bone growth and density. Pediatric patients with osteoporosis require a multidisciplinary approach that includes not only measures to strengthen bones but also to monitor and manage the underlying conditions effectively. Collaboration among pediatricians, endocrinologists, and nutritionists is essential to develop a well-rounded treatment plan that supports both bone health and overall wellbeing.

Nutritional considerations also play a critical role in managing osteoporosis in the presence of chronic diseases. For instance, patients with chronic kidney disease may need to follow a specific dietary plan that limits certain nutrients, potentially impacting calcium and vitamin D intake. Ensuring an adequate nutritional foundation is key to supporting bone health while managing coexisting conditions. Patients should work closely with dietitians to create meal plans that fulfill their unique dietary needs and promote optimal bone health, considering any restrictions imposed by their chronic diseases.

Lastly, exercise is a fundamental component of osteoporosis management, but certain chronic conditions may limit the types of physical activity that are safe and effective. For example, individuals with chronic obstructive pulmonary disease (COPD) may need to adapt their exercise routines to avoid exacerbating their respiratory condition. Engaging in weight-bearing and resistance exercises is crucial for bone health, but it must be balanced with the need to manage other health concerns. Patients should consult with physical therapists or exercise physiologists who understand the nuances of osteoporosis and can design personalized exercise programs that enhance bone strength while accommodating any limitations posed by coexisting conditions.

Importance of Comprehensive Care

Comprehensive care for osteoporosis is essential for effectively managing the condition and promoting optimal bone health. Osteoporosis is not merely a single health issue; it encompasses a wide range of factors including genetics, nutrition, physical activity, and overall lifestyle. A holistic approach ensures that all these aspects are addressed, providing patients with the tools and knowledge necessary to combat the disease. By integrating various components of care, patients can achieve better outcomes, reduce the risk of fractures, and enhance their quality of life.

The importance of individualized treatment plans cannot be overstated, particularly for populations such as postmenopausal women and pediatric patients. These groups often face unique challenges when it comes to bone health. Postmenopausal women experience a significant decline in estrogen levels, which accelerates bone loss, while children with osteoporosis may have underlying conditions that require tailored interventions. Comprehensive care allows healthcare providers to customize treatment strategies, ensuring that they meet the specific needs of these diverse patient populations.

Nutrition plays a pivotal role in the management of osteoporosis, and comprehensive care incorporates dietary assessments and interventions. Adequate intake of calcium and vitamin D is crucial for bone health, and healthcare providers can offer guidance on nutrition that supports bone density. Additionally, understanding the impact of other dietary factors, such as sodium and caffeine, can help patients make informed choices that promote stronger bones. A comprehensive approach to nutrition not only addresses dietary needs but also emphasizes the importance of healthy eating habits as part of an overall osteoporosis management plan.

Exercise physiology is another critical component of comprehensive care. Regular physical activity strengthens bones and muscles, which can help prevent fractures. A well-rounded exercise program tailored to the patient's abilities can include weight-bearing exercises, resistance training, and balance activities. Healthcare professionals can work with patients to devise a safe and effective exercise regimen that mitigates the risk of falls and improves overall physical function. This holistic approach encourages patients to take an active role in their bone health, fostering a sense of empowerment and control over their condition.

Finally, comprehensive care encompasses ongoing screening and monitoring for osteoporosis. Regular assessments enable healthcare providers to track bone density changes and adapt treatment plans as necessary. Early detection of osteoporotic fractures, as well as the management of any chronic diseases affecting bone health, is vital for preventing complications. By maintaining a proactive stance on screening and diagnosis, patients can better understand their condition and make informed decisions about their health. Overall, a comprehensive approach to osteoporosis management not only improves clinical outcomes but also fosters a supportive environment where patients feel equipped to navigate their journey toward stronger bones.

Chapter 11: Osteoporotic Fractures and Rehabilitation

Understanding Osteoporotic Fractures

Understanding osteoporotic fractures is vital for patients navigating the challenges of osteoporosis.

Osteoporotic fractures occur when bones become weakened due to decreased bone density and structural deterioration, making them more susceptible to breaks from minimal trauma. These fractures typically affect areas such as the hip, spine, and wrist, and they can significantly impact mobility and quality of life. Recognizing the types and causes of these fractures is fundamental for both prevention and treatment strategies.

The mechanisms behind osteoporotic fractures are primarily linked to the body's natural aging process, hormonal changes, and lifestyle factors. In postmenopausal women, the decline in estrogen levels accelerates bone loss, increasing fracture risk. Pediatric osteoporosis, although less common, can occur due to genetic factors, nutritional deficiencies, or underlying medical conditions. For both populations, understanding individual risk factors is essential for effective management and prevention of fractures.

Nutrition plays a crucial role in maintaining bone health and preventing fractures. A diet rich in calcium and vitamin D supports bone density and overall strength. Patients should focus on incorporating dairy products, leafy greens, and fortified foods into their meals. Additionally, certain lifestyle choices, such as avoiding excessive alcohol consumption and smoking, can further reduce the risk of fractures. It is important for patients to discuss their dietary habits with healthcare providers to ensure they are meeting their nutritional needs for optimal bone health.

Osteoporosis medications and treatments are designed to help strengthen bones and reduce the risk of fractures. Bisphosphonates, hormone replacement therapy, and newer agents such as monoclonal antibodies can effectively slow down bone loss and improve bone density. Patients should have informed discussions with their healthcare providers about the benefits and potential side effects of these treatments. Regular follow-ups can help assess the effectiveness of the prescribed regimen and make necessary adjustments based on individual responses.

Rehabilitation following an osteoporotic fracture is equally important for recovery and prevention of future fractures. A comprehensive rehabilitation program may include physical therapy, strength training, and balance exercises tailored to the patient's abilities. These interventions can help restore mobility, enhance strength, and improve balance, which are critical components in reducing the risk of future falls and fractures. Patients are encouraged to engage actively in their rehabilitation process and maintain an ongoing dialogue with their healthcare team to ensure a safe and effective recovery journey.

Strategies for Rehabilitation

Rehabilitation strategies for individuals with osteoporosis are essential for enhancing bone health, improving mobility, and reducing the risk of fractures. A comprehensive rehabilitation program should be tailored to the individual's specific needs, considering factors such as age, gender, the severity of osteoporosis, and any comorbid conditions. For postmenopausal women, pediatric patients, men, and those with osteoporosis due to chronic diseases, rehabilitation can play a crucial role in managing symptoms and promoting a better quality of life. Understanding the multifaceted approach to rehabilitation can empower patients to take control of their health.

One of the primary components of rehabilitation is exercise. A carefully designed exercise program can help strengthen bones, improve balance, and enhance overall physical function. Weight-bearing exercises, such as walking, dancing, and resistance training, are particularly beneficial as they stimulate bone formation. For patients with osteoporosis, exercises should be low-impact and focus on core strength and stability to prevent falls. It's important for patients to work with healthcare professionals, such as physical therapists, to develop a safe and effective exercise regimen that takes their individual limitations into account.

Nutrition also plays a vital role in the rehabilitation process for osteoporosis patients. Adequate intake of calcium and vitamin D is crucial for bone health. Patients should be encouraged to incorporate dairy products, leafy greens, and fortified foods into their diets while also considering supplements if necessary. Nutrition education can help patients understand the importance of a balanced diet not only for bone health but also for overall well-being. In addition, managing other dietary factors, such as limiting caffeine and alcohol, can contribute positively to rehabilitation outcomes.

Medication management is another critical aspect of rehabilitation for osteoporosis patients. Various medications are available to help strengthen bones and reduce the risk of fractures. Patients should engage in ongoing discussions with their healthcare providers regarding the benefits and potential side effects of these treatments.

Compliance with prescribed medications can significantly enhance rehabilitation efforts, as stronger bones will enable patients to participate more fully in exercise programs and other rehabilitative activities. Regular monitoring and adjustments to medication regimens can optimize treatment outcomes.

Lastly, addressing psychosocial factors is essential in the rehabilitation of osteoporosis patients. Fear of falling and sustaining fractures can hinder participation in daily activities and exercise. Psychological support, including counseling and support groups, can help patients build confidence and resilience. Additionally, patient education about osteoporosis and its management can demystify the condition, allowing individuals to actively participate in their rehabilitation. By combining physical, nutritional, and emotional support, patients can develop a holistic approach to managing osteoporosis, leading to improved outcomes and a better quality of life.

Preventing Future Fractures

Preventing future fractures is a crucial aspect of managing osteoporosis and maintaining bone health. Patients with osteoporosis are at a heightened risk of fractures, particularly in the hip, spine, and wrist. Understanding the multifaceted approaches to prevention is essential for reducing this risk. This subchapter will explore lifestyle modifications, dietary considerations, medication adherence, exercise regimens, and ongoing monitoring, all of which contribute to a comprehensive strategy for fracture prevention.

One of the most effective ways to prevent future fractures is through lifestyle modifications. Patients should focus on eliminating or minimizing risk factors such as smoking and excessive alcohol consumption, both of which can contribute to bone density loss. Additionally, creating a safe home environment is imperative. Simple changes, such as removing tripping hazards, installing grab bars in bathrooms, and ensuring adequate lighting, can significantly reduce the risk of falls that lead to fractures. Engaging in regular health check-ups can also help identify potential issues before they become serious concerns.

Nutrition plays a pivotal role in bone health, and ensuring adequate intake of essential nutrients is fundamental. Calcium and vitamin D are particularly important for maintaining bone density. Patients should aim to consume calcium-rich foods, such as dairy products, leafy greens, and fortified foods. Vitamin D, which aids in calcium absorption, can be obtained through sunlight exposure and dietary sources like fatty fish and fortified cereals. For those with specific dietary restrictions, supplements may be necessary to meet these nutritional needs. Consulting with a healthcare provider or a dietitian can help tailor a nutrition plan that aligns with individual health requirements.

Medication adherence is another critical component in preventing future fractures. For patients diagnosed with osteoporosis, medications such as bisphosphonates, hormone therapy, or newer agents like denosumab can help improve bone density and reduce the risk of fractures. It is essential for patients to understand their prescribed treatment plans and the importance of consistent medication use. Regular communication with healthcare providers about any side effects or concerns can lead to timely adjustments in treatment, maximizing the effectiveness of osteoporosis management.

Incorporating a tailored exercise regimen can significantly enhance bone strength and overall physical stability. Weight-bearing and resistance exercises are particularly beneficial for building bone density and improving balance, thus reducing the risk of falls. Patients should work with healthcare providers or physical therapists to develop a safe and effective exercise program that considers their individual capabilities and limitations. Additionally, ongoing monitoring through regular screening can help assess bone density changes and guide adjustments in prevention strategies, ensuring that patients remain proactive in their approach to bone health.